More Vignettes of Yvette at Vi

a love story of a husband for his wife

by
JOHN G. GURLEY

AuthorHouse™ LLC
1663 Liberty Drive
Bloomington, IN 47403
www.authorhouse.com
Phone: 1-800-839-8640

Published by AuthorHouse 05/15/2014

ISBN: 978-1-4969-1265-7 (sc)
978-1-4969-1264-0 (e)

Library of Congress Control Number: 2014908893

This book is printed on acid-free paper.

authorHOUSE®

INTRODUCTION

A short while ago, I wrote a little book, Vignettes of Yvette at Vi. I am now offering More Vignettes of Yvette at Vi, which I hope will add to an understanding of how to make life more interesting, enjoyable, meaningful, and even healthful for dementia sufferers. It doesn't have to be downhill all the way for these victims of Alzheimer's disease.

Carmen Galindo, Marcela Montalvo, and I care for my wife, Yvette, at the Care Center's Memory Support unit. The

Care Center is part of, and next door to, the retirement home called Vi at Palo Alto. We are on Stanford University land, and across a busy street from the Stanford Shopping Center. Memory Support has superb nurses like Rena, Marlin, Eugene, Jarvy, Lama, and others, as well as many dedicated and skilled CNAs on duty around the clock – Maria and Ernesto have been particularly helpful in caring for Yvette. Carmen, Marcela, and I are thankful that Yvette has been in such caring and capable hands.

Carmen has been, above everyone else, my main support for almost two years now. I have, in fantasy, adopted her as my granddaughter. She was born in Buenos Aires, came to this country as a university graduate student, and currently lives with her mother and a younger brother in Atherton, not far from the Care Center.

These Vignettes can stand on their own. They would, however, be better appreciated and carry more messages to the reader if the previous Vignettes were read first.

1

FROM STUPIDITY TO FELICITY

I made what I considered at the time to be a horrible mistake. It really threatened to mess up my life. Then, a few years later, it became the best move I had ever made.

I was drafted into the armed forces in 1942, several months after the attack on Pearl Harbor. After basic training at Fort Ord in California, I was sent to Brookings, South Dakota, to a cryptography school. I loved this challenge and proved so good at it that, on the basis of final examinations, I placed first in my class. I was eagerly looking forward to a career in the army of working to break enemy codes and enjoying every minute of it. Then I made the decision that put me from first place to dead last.

Each of the top students in the cryptography school was scheduled for an interview with an army officer. We guessed this was to test our overall competence to be assigned to a sensitive security position. Our loyalty to our country was to be determined. When my turn came, I entered the room, saluted my Captain, and was told to be seated. Then, rather quickly, and a surprise to me, I was confronted with the question of how I felt about Joseph Stalin and the Soviet Union. I was being asked that in September of 1942, and Hitler had invaded the Soviet Union in June of the previous year. The battle for Stalingrad was just getting underway. Officially our enemy was Hitler and one of

our allies was the Soviet Union. However, I guessed that I was
expected to answer that I had great reservations about Stalin and
his country, and even distrusted them. I thought as quickly as I
could, but my hesitation may have sealed my fate. I do not
know. Then it was definitely sealed when I decided to say what I
really believed -- that I admired many things about the Soviet
Union, our ally, and hoped they would wipe Hitler off the map.
That did it. I went from the top of the class to the bottom.

The next day, we all gathered in the auditorium for the
presentation of honors and awards. My name was not
mentioned. A few days later, I found that I had been assigned as
a clerk-typist to the Army Air Force at the Fairfield-Suisun
airbase, in California. A menial job awaited me instead of the
exalted and exciting one of cryptographer. Also our location
suggested an immediate overseas assignment into the Japanese

war zone. What had I done? I kept telling myself that I should have gotten better prepared. I might have lied. Why was I so surprised by that question? I knew that, while the Soviets were our temporary allies, they were considered in Washington to be the real enemy in the longer run.

Still, on the plus side, for the time being, I was only an hour or so from my home in Sacramento, where my parents were still living. Near my home was the tennis club that claimed most of my youthful time. I won many trophies there and made most of my friends on those courts. After a time, from Fairfield-Suisun, I got an occasional weekend pass, hitch-hiked back and forth, saw my parents, and played lots of tennis.

Nothing happened. I clerked and typed away day after day. Rumor after rumor circled the airbase. We were going to

Hawaii. No, it was Attu in the Aleutians. No, we were going to get right in the thick of it in the south seas. In the meantime, we stayed put. More typing in Fairfield-Suisun, more filing, more forms to fill out. I clerk-typed my way through the rest of 1942, all of 1943, most of 1944-- all in, what many of us began to call, that torrid war-zone near the Sacramento valley.

Then, in early October, 1944, I got another weekend pass. That Sunday morning I headed for our tennis club. And there I met Yvette, with whom I fell in love before that day was done. She came there with a tennis pal of mine, who thought that I should meet her. Yvette had graduated from San Diego State University in 1943, joined IBM and was sent to Endicott, New York, to a "computer" school. She graduated in early 1944 as an IBM machine analyst, and was then assigned to Sacramento to help maintain the State of California's huge punch-card machines that were lodged in two spacious rooms of a government building. Currently, she was living at the Senator Hotel, awaiting an apartment in a very tight wartime housing market.

When my tennis pal introduced Yvette to me, I got her first name, but her last name seemed complicated and foreign, and I never did make it out. Yvette left in the afternoon for downtown Sacramento and her hotel. That night, at dinner, I told my parents that I was going downtown to find Yvette. At the hotel, I asked at the desk if they had an Yvette. No last name, of course. The clerk told me that without a last name it would be a chore to search for her. But I was in uniform, a staff sergeant, which might have convinced him to make the effort. Yes, indeed, there was an Yvette. Full name: Yvette Magagnosc. I wrote it down, still uncertain how to pronounce it, for I did not trust the clerk's attempt.

When I saw Yvette come down to the lobby to join me, I knew for sure I was in love. The wonder to me was that Yvette felt the same way. During the next several months, I got to Sacramento as often as I could, and we were married in my parents' home on March 25, 1945. I had a 3-day pass that provided for a short honeymoon for us in Carmel. We kept our marriage as secret as we could, for IBM at that time did not employ married women. They fired any single-woman employee who got married.

I can tell you now, after 69 years of marriage, that meeting Yvette at that tennis club on that Sunday morning in October, 1944 was the most wonderful event in my life. If I had not screwed up in that interview with the Captain two years before, I never, never would have known the girl who has made my life a dream.

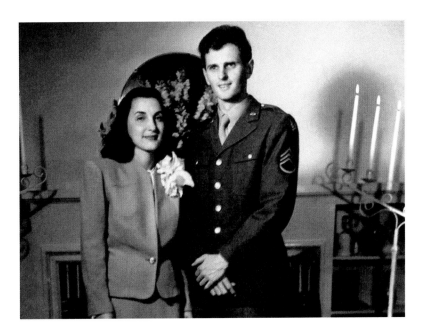

Yvette and Jack, just married

2

"I WANT TO GO HOME"

Every once in a while, like a few weeks ago when we were seated at our table in the covered plaza of La Baguette, in the Stanford Shopping Center, Yvette will say: "I want to go home." When I hear that, my heart nearly stops, and a great sadness comes over me, even though I do not know exactly what Yvette means.

She cannot mean the apartment I am currently living in and that we together occupied for seven years. She never liked our move from our campus home to this retirement home. When we got here, Yvette found that she was unable to operate any of the appliances -- the dishwasher, clothes washer and dryer, the stove, or its oven. All the knobs were different and strangely placed. Even how to open the refrigerator door baffled her. She knew her appliances in our campus home as long-time friends, but now all of these new ones were foes. It never occurred to me at that time that I was witnessing my wife in the early stages of dementia. I kept trying to show her how, but I soon found myself absorbed in preparing our meals, and before much longer doing everything else necessary to keep a household going. Yvette, of course, hated her demotion, wanted to help but could not. No, this isn't the home Yvette has in mind when she tells me "I want to go home."

She might have in mind our Stanford campus home, which Yvette and I lived in for 44 years, and which she helped to design architecturally. This was a home that Yvette loved. And yet, a few years ago, just before she had to go to Memory Support, when I drove her past our campus home, she didn't seem to have much interest in it. Since Yvette has been in Memory Support, I have frequently mentioned our campus home, describing our garden room with the fountain in the middle of it, our living room that was equally our library, with many shelves for our books, her super kitchen that had a center island and views of the fountain in the garden room, and much more. Yvette listens but fails to react in any way that suggests she really misses that home. Still, I may be misreading her and she may have this home in mind when she tells me about wanting to go home. I honestly do not know.

It is possible that she is referring to the last home she lived in with her parents, before she left for the university, which was at Lake Elsinore, halfway between Los Angeles and San Diego. Many dementia patients, we are told, retain vivid long-term memories, so Yvette may be reaching way back to this home.

It is also possible that she means nothing definite by her wish. It's simply something she says. When I hear Yvette say she wants to go home, I try to recover my composure by supposing she means nothing by it. She's just talking. But in the back of my mind is the disturbing thought that, while she may have no particular home in mind, Yvette is telling us that she does not like it in Memory Support. "I want to go home," means "I want to get out of here." No destination in mind, just don't hold me in here any longer. A few moments later, however,

Yvette is laughing at the antics of a little girl, who is chasing a

pigeon. Then, I relax -- until the next time.

Now, let me tell you about the next time. It was this

afternoon, again at La Baguette, when Yvette suddenly said:

"Maybe eventually I can go home." This suggested some

understanding of her need right now to be in Memory Support,

but that "eventually" she might be able to go home. "Maybe"

eventually -- there was some uncertainty there. And that from

someone with dementia, who has been under care in Memory

Support for two years. I looked at Yvette, my dear and lovely

wife of 69 years, and I held her hand and did everything I could

to keep from crying.

3

WALKING AND TALKING

About the time that Yvette could no longer walk, she also stopped talking. This occurred in Memory Support, after a year there.

She wanted to keep walking, but she was no longer getting adequate instructions from her brain on how to do it. During the period of declining mobility, there were many falls from tripping over nothing that I could see. Then Yvette began having trouble in positioning herself to sit down on a chair or sofa. More and more, she needed our help. Getting up, after sitting down, became increasingly difficult. Her brain was letting her down, if I may express it so. Finally, just trying to walk proved too much, and Carmen and I ordered a transport chair for Yvette. We quickly learned that dementia often has as many physical ramifications as mental.

Someone in authority advised me to accept it willingly, for in a chair Yvette would not fall again. She would easily get used to it. Anyway, she's probably not going to walk again, so get her comfortable in her chair and plan excursions for her. If you look around Memory Support, and you've been over there as frequently as I have, this would seem to you like wise counsel. Many of the 24 residents in the two Memory Support units are in wheelchairs, and once there, always there. In those units, no-one goes from wheelchair back to walking again.

However, Carmen, from the very beginning, did not accept this as inevitable for Yvette. Every morning, before Yvette was helped out of bed, Carmen would massage Yvette's legs, and then, holding her feet, would flex her legs as though she were on a bicycle. During some part of each day, Carmen encouraged Yvette to use her feet to move the transport chair backwards and forwards. Actually, Yvette soon came to love this activity, and was continually trying to free one foot from her foot rests so as to back-pedal her chair, wherever she happened to be. Yvette does this with her left foot only, for she still favors her right foot which had a wound that took a long time to heal. Although the wound is now completely gone, Yvette still does not trust that foot.

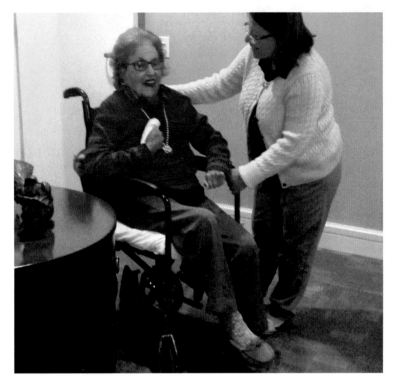

Back-pedaling with Carmen

Then, Carmen and I heard about bicycle pedals that could be placed on the floor and used by Yvette while she was in her chair. Two days later, Amazon delivered them, and ever since Yvette has exercised with them at least half an hour each day.

Yvette seemingly likes these pedals and never has to be urged or forced to use them. When she does pedal, she is exercising both legs, instead of just the left when back-pedaling.

Finally, every day Carmen gets another staff member to help her get Yvette out of her chair and onto her feet. Then, Yvette, between the two, walks with them as far as she can. She then gets back into the chair. Yvette back-pedals the chair to return to the starting gate, as we call it, and is ready again for more walking. My job is to wheel the chair behind Yvette for her to use when she tires. That may seem to be a menial task, but it does require close attention to Yvette's rear end, to see whether it is sagging. If it is, I get her chair under her fast. So far I've had no complaints about my performances.

So what do we think we're doing? We have in mind that Yvette, before much longer, is going to walk using a walker. Her legs are getting stronger, she is walking "lighter" with her two aides as time goes on, she can now rise from the toilet to a standing position without using her arms, just the strength of her legs, and she wants to walk. She misses walking! Carmen and I both know that for sure. When Yvette is sitting in her chair with her feet on the foot rests, she often begins moving her legs as though she were pedaling. She clearly enjoys and wants leg exercises.

Although we have made much progress, I think we might not make it all the way to a walker. Carmen thinks we will. We both know, however, that we need to keep doing what we're doing. It simply isn't right to give up on Yvette and sentence her to the transport chair for the rest of her life, especially when

Yvette is telling us every day of her desire to walk again. We are all responding to that in the best way we know how.

Yvette stopped talking around the time that she stopped walking. The two were probably not causally related, for the walking stoppage was involuntary, while the talking stoppage was clearly voluntary. Yvette could talk all right, but her talking was becoming indistinct, so much so finally that Carmen and I made out very little of what Yvette was trying to tell us. We often did not respond to what we did not understand. That seemed to discourage Yvette so very deeply as to lead her to stop talking altogether. This silence lasted for many, many weeks.

Finally, Carmen and I agreed that we had to do something about that. We began to ask Yvette to respond to whatever we were telling or asking her. What do you think? Would you like that? How are you feeling? Are you hungry, thirsty? Carmen and I made remarks to each other meant to provoke Yvette into saying something. I talked about my sister, Helen, about her dog, Taj, about anything funny that had recently happened. After weeks of this, just as we were beginning to get discouraged, Yvette decided to talk again.

Carmen and I were prepared. We pretended to understand everything Yvette said. She spoke. If we did not understand, we replied "oh, yes?" Yvette responded "yes," as though she were saying "I meant what I said." We actually understood some of what Yvette said. Then more. We never failed to respond to her. These tactics induced Yvette to talk more and more, and we began understanding some wonderful and clear statements. "Have a seat," she said to me as we entered the family room together. "He's my husband," she said to Carmen, indicating me. That put me in seventh Heaven. "ATM," she said clearly, reading a sign some distance away. That one served also to tell us something about her eyes and glasses, information we could not get otherwise. It also told us she was looking around, focusing on distant things.

This morning Yvette looked beautiful, after Carmen and Maria showered her, and Carmen dressed her in lovely, matching clothes. Once Yvette is in her transport chair she is likely to say "Let's go." However, this morning, she came out with a more complete sentence, saying clearly: "Let's go for a walk." She got kisses from both of us. In return, we got a gorgeous smile, which, I think, was not only for our kisses, but also for her own vocal performance. She had a perfect right to be proud of herself. Just consider how much preparation that must have required.

Then we had a major breakthrough. "Look at her," Yvette said. "I know her." "I didn't see her," I said. "I did," Yvette replied. Two things there bowled us over. First, Yvette made two statements in a row. Second, she responded to my reply. That, my friends, was a conversation, the first between us in over a year. In recent weeks, Yvette has not only been talking more, but, as I just noted, she is now responding to our replies to what she first said -- which gave us more pleasure and satisfaction than I can express. We told Yvette how wonderful that all was, and she replied to that, too, with a smile and then a laugh.

So Carmen and I believe our efforts have been successful in getting Yvette to talk more and more, in more complex ways, and with increasingly more things said clearly. We are thrilled with every articulated word from her. That's the talking part. The walking part may be a different beast, but Carmen has often chided me for saying things like that. Still, we have made great progress. I know that Yvette wants us to work hard at getting her back walking again. I will certainly and gladly do what I can. None of us is going to let Yvette down.

4

SLEEPY-HEAD

For Yvette, the Sleep Fairy accompanies the Dementia Beast through the halls of Memory Support. Unlike other sufferers from this disease, who have sleep disorders, Yvette has been sleeping soundly and long. She generally gets 12 hours of sleep each night. She has a nap in the morning from 9:45 to 11:00. In the afternoon, she naps from 1:45 to 3:00. So we add 2 1/2 hours to the 12 and get 14 1/2 hours of sleep out of 24 hours, or 60 per cent. Yvette is awake only 40 per cent of the time. We do not have to add to this the time she is awake trying to go to sleep. Once she is settled in bed, for the night or for naps, she is sound asleep in 15 seconds. I think the Sleep Fairy has a soft brush that she uses to dab Yvette's eyelids with a heavenly lotion -- and, bango, Yvette is in the sleep world. Dementia, with the aid of the Sleep Fairy, decided to make Yvette a sleepy-head.

When Carmen arrives in the morning to awaken Yvette, sometimes she is only half asleep. When she hears somebody enter her room, Yvette opens her eyes to see who it is. Then she quickly closes them to pretend she is still sound asleep. But there is a tell-tale sign. If Yvette is really awake, her left hand, now in the form of a fist, begins rapid movements in preparation for an upper-cut to the jaw of anyone even thinking of getting her up. Another tell-tale sign that Yvette has sighted enemy forces near her bed is the tightening of her lips. Her eyelids may still be closed, but those about to enter combat are not fooled. It requires combat-ready troops to hold Yvette to only 14 1/2 hours of sleep each day.

I often wonder just how long Yvette would sleep each day if she was not forced three times daily into combat. My first quick and useless answer is longer. But consider this: Yvette may be laughing and quite awake when we decide it is time for her nap. In 15 seconds, she is in bed. In another 15 seconds, she is sound asleep. Aren't we forcing sleep on her? So, really, I'm not sure how many hours she would sleep in the absence not only of enemy forces but also of the friendly forces that put her to bed. When I have the chance, I shall ask the Sleep Fairy.

5

BURRITOS

Several months ago, Yvette's fingers began to curl up into fists. They are not really tight fists, but no-one would fail to see them as fists. This prevented her from doing all sorts of things. She could not shake hands with anyone wanting to do that. She could not perform many bathroom duties. She could not pick up anything. This last meant that she was no longer able to feed herself, for the handling of utensils was out. She was unable to grasp a glass for a drink of water. Well, I needn't go on, for all you have to do is think of all the uses you make of your open

hands throughout the day.

When Carmen saw what was happening, she rolled up a

bathroom wash cloth into a cylindrical shape and forced it into

Yvette's right hand. Yvette seemingly did not mind holding it --

or its replacements -- throughout the day and night. Yvette is

left-handed, so Carmen let her use her loose left fist for threats,

"holding hands," caressing someone's cheek, or anything else.

At night, however, Yvette often holds two of what Carmen

began to call "burritos."

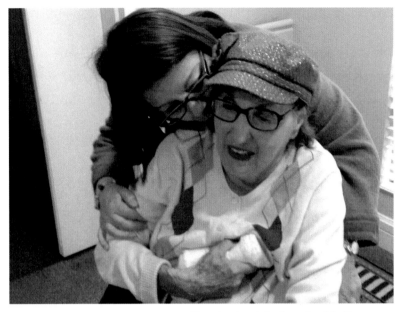

Burrito in right hand, with Carmen

The burritos serve several purposes. They tell Yvette that if she can hold a burrito perhaps she can hold a glass of water. And indeed Carmen, a few times, has guided Yvette into just that. When Yvette hangs on to a burrito for hour after hour, it also helps to prevent her fingers from curling up even more. Moreover, burritos keep Yvette's fingers from continually rubbing the palm of her hand, which reduces skin damage. The burritos absorb much of the odors that arise from a clenched fist held that way all day. The burritos can be changed and the old ones washed. They are sometimes the talk of the town. "What in the world is Yvette holding in her right hand?" "It's a burrito". "A what?" "A burrito." "Well, I never . . ."

Yvette holds on to a burrito in her right hand 24 hours a day, and for a lesser time in her left hand. The Dementia Beast, and Carmen's ingenuity, have made burritos a necessary part of what Yvette now is. We wrack our brains day by day, hoping to keep the Beast at bay.

6

SANITATION WORKERS

The people at the Shopping Center, who seem to have the greatest interest in Yvette, are the sanitation workers, men and women. These are the workers who clean out the trash cans, put new plastic bags in the cans, and sweep and sweep from one end of the mall to the other, and then back. Their interest in us is probably because they are always there and see Yvette, Carmen, and me almost daily. Also, they all speak Spanish and enjoy conversing with Carmen in their own language. A few have told us how much they admire the warm relationship they have observed between Yvette and me. Several got to know us when

we were ministering to the ailing pigeon, Bernadette. By now,

they have become our good friends, and all have received copies

of the Bernadette booklet and of my book, Vignettes of Yvette at

Vi. They have gone out of their way to tell us how much they

enjoyed those stories. Carmen and I treasure their friendship.

Yvette doesn't know it, but we have been told that her beautiful

attire played a role in attracting them to us in the first place.

7

HELLO, STRANGER

On some of our walks through the Stanford Shopping

Center, with Carmen or Marcela, Yvette will hold out her hand

to people passing the other way, and say "Hello." That's her left

hand, which is in the form of a fist because that is what her brain

is telling her fingers to do. Some of the passers-by, seeing that

fist pointing straight at them, might believe that they are being

challenged to a boxing match. But as the arm and fist go out,

Yvette is saying "Hello." That usually results in a double-take by the passers-by, and some of them stop, go over to Yvette to say "Hello," and to tell her how pretty she looks.

Today was such a day. Yvette, with her fist and voice, was greeting almost everyone coming the other way. At one point, she greeted a man, whose dog, on a leash, was getting a drink from a metal bowl in front of the Microsoft store. The man's attention turned to Yvette, and he was starting to come over, but his dog, having quenched his thirst, would not budge. Finally, the man shrugged and told us that he momentarily forgot that his dog always got a cookie after having a drink right there, so he had better attend to that. We went on our way to hold out our fist to anyone else coming along. A real big "Hello," too.

8

TELLING STORIES

Carmen and I talk to Yvette every day, for hours, about recent and distant events in her life. We usually start out by telling her each day what the day of the week it is, and we try to support that by relating it to what she knows. One reference is to the number of shoppers at the Stanford Shopping Center, where we go every day. If this is Tuesday, we do not see many shoppers and there are hardly any children. We tell Yvette that on Tuesdays we never see the crowds we see on weekends. Also Tuesday is a school day, so that's why there are so few children here today. To get to the Shopping Center, we must cross Sand Hill Road, a busy street. We always relate the amount of traffic to the day of the week. There seem to be few cars today, Yvette, but that's because today is Sunday. Then, a few minutes later, we are among masses of Sunday shoppers. You see, Yvette, it is Sunday. Look at all these shoppers. Oh, Yvette, have you ever seen so many dogs? That works for Yvette because she knows the dogs show up on Sundays. And she knows that because she has heard it from us many times and has seen it while we are talking about it. I think that Yvette is au courant on days of the week.

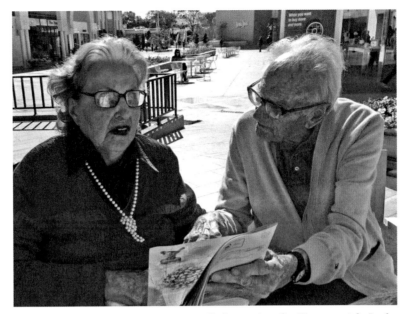

Information for Yvette, with Jack

Shoppers, children, dogs, and traffic are related to days of the week. It is not difficult to find things to relate to events in Yvette's life. A passer-by who looks like someone we knew at the Brookings Institution in Washington, D.C., where we worked together for several years. Pretty dresses in a shop

window that remind me of Oscar de la Renta at Casa de Campo

in the Dominican Republic, where we spent some time. A shop

that has a branch in San Diego, where Yvette spent her

university years. Well, almost anything will do, or really nothing

at all, for me to tell Yvette stories about her days at Princeton,

her tennis matches in Bethesda, her house overlooking the

Potomac River, her days with IBM and computers. It's no big

deal to find a link to something important in Yvette's life. What

is a big deal is to tell these stories day after day in ways to keep

Yvette's attention on them. Carmen and I were not too good at

this at first, but now that we've been at it for two years, we think

we have had Yvette's attention enough to say that she does have

in mind many recent and distant events that were important to

her. It's no deep secret. You just have to keep at it.

9

BATHROOM DRAMA

When Carmen, with another aide, often male, preceding
her, wheels Yvette out of her bathroom, after she has been in
there ten to twenty minutes, and I am seated in her room
awaiting her, Yvette usually looks at me -- straight through me.
For a few minutes, she sees me and she doesn't see me. She is
stressed out. I have seen this 700 times, and not once have I seen
Yvette smiling as she emerges from what must be her bathroom
distress. That's 0 for 700. Not 1 or 2 out of 700, but zero. Do we
need another 700 observations to conclude that even those with

dementia find something very upsetting about having to go to the toilet, often with two people looking on? Yvette does not walk, she often speaks indistinctly, she has forgotten many things, but you better believe that she retains a sense of decorum, an understanding when indignities are being pressed on her. Yvette may not recognize some old friend, but she still knows when she is being embarrassed. Carmen and her helpers are in no way to blame. They always do what is best for Yvette. It's just an unfortunate situation imposed by the demands of dementia on all of them.

10

OUR SUNDAY LUNCHES

On many Sundays, Carmen and I take Yvette for lunch to the restaurant on the third floor of Neiman Marcus. We generally wait outside in the sun for a few minutes until they open the doors at noon. Then Carmen wheels Yvette toward the elevators, stopping briefly at the perfume counter for a bit more fragrance for Yvette. After getting off the elevator at the third floor, and passing through all the cute and dressy children's clothes, we are greeted enthusiastically by the hostess, and in a minute or two also by the women servers. We have "our" table where Yvette is positioned so she can see almost everyone there. Carmen sits on Yvette's right, and I on her left.

Our lunch is like something you've never seen before. Yvette can eat only by being fed by Carmen, because her fingers on each hand are curled up into fists, preventing her from handling utensils. That means that Yvette eats her lunch first, before Carmen and I eat ours. Carmen is busy feeding Yvette, but I have nothing to do, so I'm idling in neutral. I do have a popover and iced tea, so I break the popover into a hundred little pieces and eat them as slowly as I can.

Since her bout with aspiration pneumonia, Yvette is eating only puréed food, so our best bet is to order a large bowl of hearty soup for her. On this Sunday, the restaurant had lentil and pork soup, and in the kitchen they gladly put it in a blender and puréed it for Yvette. Then with a small spoon, Carmen goes to work. This generally takes thirty to forty minutes, for Yvette is, as usual, eating slowly and thoroughly enjoying her food. Halfway through Yvette's lunch, we order ours, usually salads, which are ready for us when Yvette has finished.

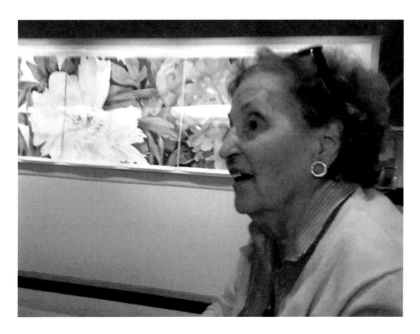

Yvette at Sunday Lunch, Neiman Marcus

Now what does Yvette do while we are eating our salads? When she is at any dining table, Yvette is quiet, sits regally like a queen, and appears to be looking over her subjects. There is a lot to look at in this restaurant. However, Carmen or I always order a salad that has avocados, for these in small pieces Yvette can eat as puréed food. So Carmen can't eat entirely in peace, but has to give Yvette every now and then some avocado pieces. This requires moving her chair over to Yvette, and then back again when she resumes eating. It's lucky no one is really watching us. No-one seems to be saying: "Did you see that?"

The women servers, of course, know what's going on. When they are able to, they always come over to chat with us and to say some nice things to Yvette. They have read my books on Bernadette and Yvette, so they know all about us. They have been our friends for some time now, which is one good reason why we keep showing up.

Just this afternoon, the young woman who always starts us off at Sunday lunch with popovers came upon us while we were seated at La Baguette, rushed up to give Yvette a hug and kiss, then the same for Carmen and me. It is so enjoyable for us, when we are with Yvette, to see her treated so lovingly by others.

11

BEAUTY AND THE BEAST

There is no reason at all to sacrifice Beauty simply because the Beast of Dementia has its claws around you. Beauty should not only live on but be enhanced, thereby really defying the Beast. It is a shame that so many dementia sufferers, by the neglect of family and friends, are sent into a decline in dress and appearance -- or, at best, are saddled with the same wardrobe month after month after month. Carmen, from the beginning, thumbed her nose at the Beast, and presented Yvette as Beauty Enhanced each and every day.

The wardrobe that Yvette brought with her when she entered Memory Support was already fairly nice. She had more than a dozen dress shirts by Faconnable in Paris, more than that number in sweaters, a few from Yves St. Laurent, many from Land's End, and a couple from Max Mara. There were pants of many hues to match the shirts and sweaters. Colorful socks and comfortable sandals and shoes were also included. Finally, Yvette had many -- probably too many-- necklaces, and there were some very attractive scarves.

Carmen added earrings, which Yvette had never worn, and, as time went on, kept altering the wardrobe with new things. Several beautiful scarves were added, an elegant black and white shirt-sweater from Brooks Brothers, half a dozen classy hats with visors from Macy's, a lovely sweater from Nordstrom's, moccasins with soft wool inside, more pants from Land's End, and yet additional shirts from Bloomingdale's. In this way,

Yvette was presented daily as a Beauty and so was announcing

that no Beast was going to put her into a sartorial tailspin. The

Beast may have placed her in a transport chair, but, by all the

gods, she was going to look pretty in it.

Carmen has a sharp eye for pleasing combinations of attire.

A pink stripe, for example, in a shirt sporting other colors, too,

might call for a matching pink sweater. That theme is then

carried down to the socks, and, if called for, to a gorgeous scarf.

Yvette's hair is attended to on Monday mornings at the Beauty

Salon in the Care Center. Carmen keeps her hair looking good

the rest of the week. Every day Carmen is taunting the Beast

with sartorial splendor and attractive hairdos on her Beauty.

Take that, you beastly Beast -- and that! And then earrings and a

necklace will really show that creature!

In "dress and appearance," that's the dress and part of the appearance. The other part of appearance concerns what is underneath the attire, and that calls for washing, showering, applied body lotions, sprays, as well as, at the end, facial makeup. Even after all that, when Carmen is wheeling Yvette through Macy's, there is always a stop at a perfume counter for a bit more fragrance. The Beast by this time, doesn't know what hit him!

For her age, Yvette is a pretty lady anyway. However, Carmen knows how easy it would be just to give in to the Beast and let Yvette's natural good-looks get her by. Shower her a few times a week, throw on any clothes, forget new items to the wardrobe, use what you have, let her hair go gray, toss away the lipstick and powder. No. Carmen knows the Beast is there, and she is determined to keep it at bay, day after day, with dazzling

Beauty displays.

It is love for Yvette that generates that much care at the

Care Center.

12

GIGI AND ELLA MARIE

Gigi and Ella Marie are the latest arrivals to Memory Support 2. Their presence has lowered the average age of the dementia residents plus these two newcomers by many years, for Gigi is only 3 months old, and Ella Marie is just 3 months older than that. Gigi is the granddaughter of Lindsay Morgenthaler, who is in MS 2 with Yvette. Ella Marie is the granddaughter of Irma Lomeli, a Server in the Bistro restaurant in Vi, and whose daughter-in-law, Ana Cecilia Quijano, a staff member in Activities at the Care Center, is the mother.

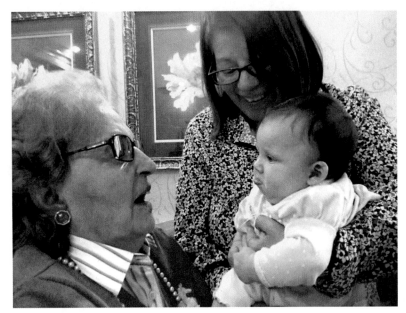

Gigi and Yvette with Carmen

Cute Ella Marie is brought in only occasionally, but Gigi

seems to be there, with her nanny, almost every day. Gigi is

passed around from one person to another. Carmen loves to hold

her, and she has introduced Gigi many times to Yvette. A

picture that I took of one of the earlier meetings seems to show

that neither Yvette nor Gigi had quite figured out the other. A later photo, however, suggests that they now seem to like each other very much. When Yvette today was shown the second picture, she said with a big smile: "That is my little friend." That was a wonderful, complete sentence for Yvette, and it made Carmen and me so pleased with the progress Yvette has made in talking to us. Let's give Gigi a big assist.

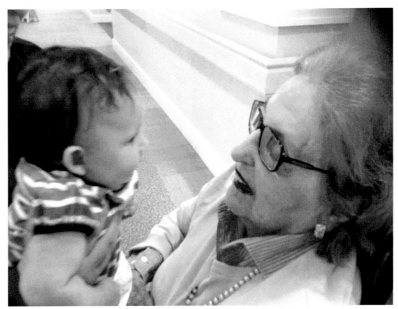

That is my little friend

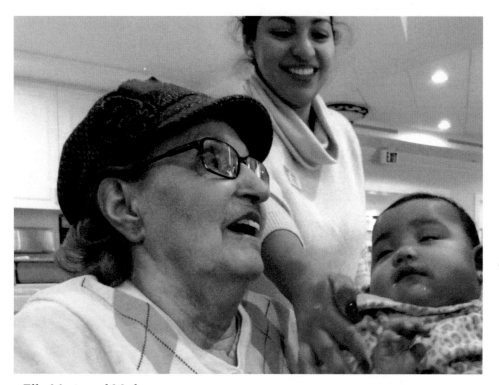

Ella Marie and Mother

13

PARTY TIME

In an earlier Vignette, I mentioned the Stanford friends of Yvette who went missing when Yvette went into Memory Support at the Care Center. Two years later, Carmen decided to round up some of them for a party to celebrate Yvette's and my 69th wedding anniversary. Carmen pulled off this roundup, without my knowledge, through Edythe Hickman; she and her family lived across the street from us on the Stanford campus, and are now residents at Vi.

Carmen and I had previously purchased a new outfit for Yvette for this occasion -- an elegant green sweater with a pleated undershirt just showing above the sweater's V. A pearl necklace, white pants, sparkling shoes, pretty earrings, and socks out of this world completed the ensemble.

Yvette was more than ready sartorially. But I was fearful that Yvette, not relishing crowds these past two years, would greet her guests with fidgeting and loud vocal sounds and would not enjoy herself. If I had known about the great roundup, I would have had further concerns -- about whether Yvette would recognize her old friends after not seeing some of them for at least two years. Would she even open her eyes to look at them? Yes, all dressed up, but perhaps mentally down.

Party time. Nine Stanford friends arrived, five of whom Yvette had not seen for a long while. Other guests came, too, including two servers at the restaurant in Neiman Marcus, one with her entire family, and the other with a chocolate cake. Several of the staff of Memory Support dropped in from time to time. Gigi, her mother, Lissa, and nanny came with a beautiful card for us. We had, at any one time, about twenty people in the Family Room of MS 1, a room we call the Women's' Gym. Now it was Party Headquarters, with sandwiches and a variety of snacks, soft drinks, and a magnificent strawberry cake to come.

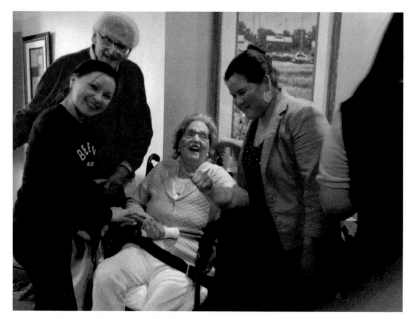

Friends from our Sunday Lunch, Neiman Marcus

I am so very happy to be wrong, both in what I said and in

what I thought. I said in a previous Vignette that Yvette during

her first year in Memory Support was fast forgetting her friends.

She gave every indication, as they arrived at the Party, of

remembering them, giving each a big smile, with some

prompting calling one by her name, and actually carrying on

brief conversations with a few. Once when I told Yvette that
Dorothy Anderson had just come in, Yvette said: "I know." I
believed her. Also I thought, probably feared, that she would
give her usual signs of agitation, unhappy with so many people
around her, and not enjoy what Carmen had planned for her.
Wrong, wrong, wrong. Yvette was all smiles from start to finish.
I have not seen her so happy for that length of time since she
entered Memory Support.

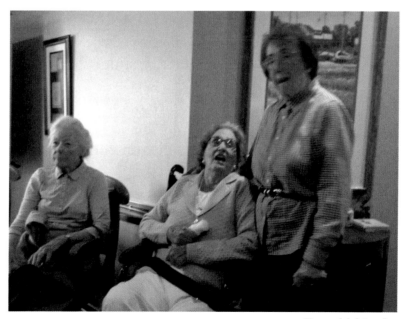

Two old friends

What a contrast with last year's celebration! Then Yvette slept through most of it, never smiled, looked out of it. Maybe three things can explain this big difference. Most important was the medication -- the tranquilizer -- she was taking. This seemed to have two seemingly incompatible effects -- drowsiness and aggression, the latter not only against others but also against herself. We quickly got rid of the tranquilizer. Also her Stanford friends were not there, which may account for some of the lesser interest she had in that first party. Finally, Carmen and I believe that, during the past year, we have stimulated Yvette with our daily discussions of the major events in her life, our reminders of what's going on each day, and our constant attempts to get her to talk more. She seems more alert much of the time. She has, without question, improved substantially in this regard over a year ago.

When I suggested to Yvette a few days ago that we might go outside later and look at the moonlight (we had just listened to Beethoven's Moonlight Sonata), her response was "baloney." If I had suggested that a year ago, she most likely would not have heard me, or, having heard me, would have had nothing to say. I consider "baloney" a gigantic step forward.

14

ROOM FOR COLOR

When I knew that Yvette would have to move over to Memory Support, I had no time to purchase furniture, so I quickly decided that I would rent some for a brief interval that would give me time to think about what to buy. As it turned out, I made two errors "on one ground ball to the infield": what I rented was far from ideal, and I kept it much too long.

I rented an easy chair, a short sofa, a chest of drawers, and a corner table. In the abstract those were okay. But the chair and sofa were too large, bulky, and really dull looking -- browns and tans. The other pieces were dark browns. We managed to fit them all in the room -- along with a bed and an armoire (another brown), both supplied by Memory Support. As a consequence, the room looked small, there wasn't much space left to move around, and it's hard to imagine how drab and dreary the whole thing was. In the early months, not really aware of the room's drabness, I must have, almost unconsciously, tried to brighten things up with pictures on the walls. Yvette, for a long time, has liked the French Impressionists, so we have many reproductions of their paintings. I used some of these, especially Monets and Renoirs, and in addition a Mary Cassatt and a Van Gogh, to give some life to the room. But I really wasn't thinking that I had to do this because of the deadly furniture.

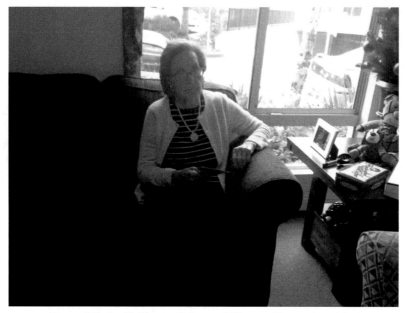

Rented Sofa, Table, and Arm of Chair, Christmas, 2012.

Carmen and I were so involved with other things having to do with Yvette that we never even had time to assess or discuss the decor of her room. I paid the rental fee month after month without thinking about it. I let almost two years go by before I realized that Yvette was living in a space with over-stuffed, bulging, and uninspiring furniture. Browns and tans everywhere.

"Let's get some color in there," I said to Carmen one recent afternoon. "And," I added, "let's see if we can downsize. That will make the room seem larger." Carmen agreed, but she had no time for this business, so it was up to me.

Since I get almost everything, even my shoelaces and toothpaste, from Amazon these days, why not furniture? Amazon, old pal, do you have an easy chair, not too big, with reds, oranges, and blues, also yellows and greens, all over it? While we're at it, dot com, how about the same in a small sofa, a loveseat? After days and days of repeatedly running my iPad's batteries to zero, our friend, Amazon, gave us the clues to find just what we wanted -- but not from Amazon.

Now I'm faced with logistics. If the new stuff comes in before the old stuff goes out, where am I going to store the new stuff. I'm in an apartment, independent living, while Yvette is in

Memory Support. We don't want the old stuff out too soon, days

before the new stuff gets here. Part of the old stuff is a chest of

drawers, which contains in its four drawers much of Yvette's

clothes. My plan was to replace that with a Japanese chest --

also filled with Yvette's things -- that I had in my apartment.

Clothes had to be transferred from the old to the new -- but not

too soon, for there was little room for another piece of furniture

in Yvette's place.

A schedule was set for one thing, which required requests

from me for other schedules, and then the first supplier said it

would be two days later, sorry, which got me back on the phone

to the others, all the time wondering when the old stuff was ever

going to be picked up, and what was I going to do with all the

clothes I found in the Japanese chest, and would Carmen like any of them for Yvette, or should I go for a tax deduction by giving them away, a decision that was interrupted by a phone call from the old stuff that it would be five days from now, which of course got me back to the chair guy and the loveseat woman, who were ticked off, claiming I had schedulitis, a disease that would quickly spread to everyone involved in this ill-fated enterprise, necessitating a call to my tax lawyer, who managed to get the whole thing untangled and shipshape with a fee exceeding the cost of our loveseat, including shipping and tax.

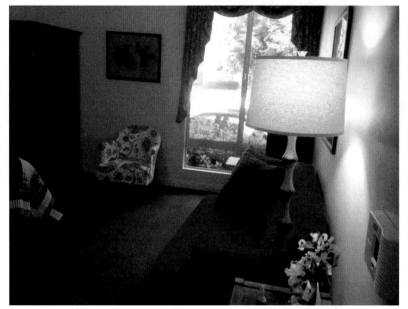

New Sofa, Lamp, Chair, Picture, and Bedspread. April, 2014.

Well, with the old stuff ausgegagen and the new stuff

ingegagen, we added a few appropriate paintings, a new

bedspread, with colors complementary to those of the furniture,

and a floor lamp. Lots of color, smaller pieces, larger-looking,

brighter room. Carmen and I believe that Yvette will gain from

this transformation, stimulated by the beauty of her new decor, just as she seems stimulated by others mentioning her own beauty. We feel that the Dementia Beast must be thwarted not only by Yvette as Beauty Enhanced but also by her room as Decor Delight. We're not giving up without a fight.

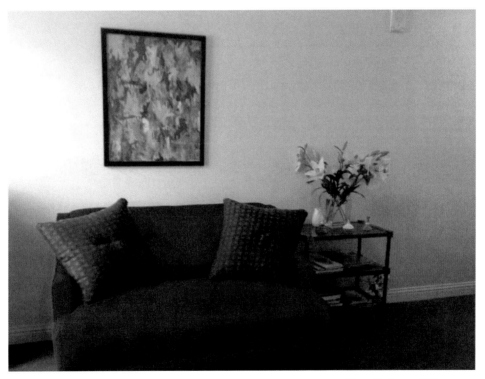

New Sofa and Picture.

15

IS YVETTE HAPPY?

Are you? That's a very difficult question for anyone to answer. For an obvious reason, I cannot ask Yvette if she's happy, but I can, day after day, watch her for smiles, listen for laughter, examine her facial expressions, note what she is saying, try to interpret her vocal sounds, and just see whether her body is relaxed or in some type of agitation.

Now, before I go on, I want to record that, in my limited experience, dementia sufferers do not smile and laugh very much. Oh yes, I've seen a few smiles in the past two years, a few pleasant looks, and some contented ones, but never a full smile that Yvette very often gives us. Laughs? Yvette frequently laughs -- and that's about it for the Memory Support units, for I have seldom observed anyone else, over two years, doing the same. People with dementia, those I've observed, generally have sober looks, or they are staring at a newspaper or TV, or more often asleep.

So I would say that Yvette has been unusual among the 30 to 35 people who have been in the Memory Support units the past two years. However, that does not mean that no one else is happy -- some may well be --and it does not even mean that Yvette herself is, on balance, happy. Certainly, the many broad smiles and the occasional laughs suggest that Yvette is happy much of the time. But there are also lengthy periods of agitation, accompanied by vocal sounds, that tell me she is not happy at other times.

Now let me add what has often broken my heart and disturbed me into the night. Yvette will look at me, directly into my eyes, and say: "I want you to save me." Or "I need help." Or "Please help me." Or "I want to go home." Not often, but enough to caution me about saying outright that she is happy. When Yvette is smiling and laughing -- and that's often enough -- she is exceptional, and Carmen, Marcela, and I rejoice. At those other, disturbing times, I wonder about my wife with dementia knowing she is in trouble. That would not seem to translate easily into happiness.

But I have come to believe that those expressions do not run deep, for, if they did, Carmen and I would have seen quite a different Yvette. We have actually seen an attractive lady very prone to smiles and laughter when she recognizes a friend, when she is observing, at La Baguette, little kids frolicking around or anything out of the ordinary, when at meal times funny things happen, when she is exercising by pedaling or moving backwards in her chair, or when she is told that we are going to "Stanford." She smiles frequently at Carmen, Marcela, and me. Those and other happy moments, however, are far from adding to a day. So, no, not fully happy, but our lovely companion is pretty happy.

16

CRAZY AS A LOVE-BIRD

Have you been wanting for some time now to call me crazy? Well, here at last is your chance. You won't have a better one, so jump on this doozy.

Every night, while alone in "our" apartment, I talk aloud to Yvette. I tell her that I hope she will have a good night's sleep. I tell her that Carmen (or Marcela) is going to dress her beautifully in the morning, that she will have a nice breakfast, and that I will see her near the end of her breakfast and then be with her for most of the day. I tell her how very much I love her.

I readily admit the craziness of all that. Of course, Yvette doesn't hear me. And yet, each night for two years I have talked to Yvette. I do it because it keeps me close to her. It keeps me going. It's the craziness of it all that keeps me sane.

Printed in the United States
By Bookmasters